Keto Migraine

A Beginner's Quick Start Guide for Women on Managing Migraines Through the Ketogenic Diet, With Sample Curated Recipes

STEPHANIE HINDEROCK

Disclaimer

By reading this disclaimer, you are accepting the terms of the disclaimer in full. If you disagree with this disclaimer, please do not use this website.

All of the content within this website is provided for informational and educational purposes only, and should not be accepted as independent medical or other professional advice. The author of these articles is not a doctor, physician, nurse, mental health provider, or registered nutritionist/dietician. Therefore, using and reading any of the content on this website does not establish any form of a physician-patient relationship.

Always consult with a physician or another qualified health provider with any issues or questions you might have regarding any sort of medical condition. Do not ever disregard any qualified professional medical advice or delay seeking that advice because of anything you have read in this guide. The information in this guide is not intended to be any sort of medical advice and should not be used in lieu of any medical advice by a licensed and qualified medical professional.

The information on this website has been compiled from a variety of known sources. However, the author cannot attest to or guarantee the accuracy of each source and thus should not be held liable for any errors or omissions.

Introduction

A migraine is a type of headache that is characterized by intense, throbbing pain. Migraines often occur with other symptoms, such as nausea, vomiting, and sensitivity to light. Migraines typically last for several hours and can be so severe that they interfere with daily activities.

The exact cause of migraines is not known, but they are thought to be due to changes in the brainstem and trigeminal nerve. This theory is supported by the fact that migraines often run in families.

Treatment for migraines typically involves taking pain relievers or anti-inflammatory drugs. Some people also find relief from wearing dark glasses and lying down in a quiet, darkened room. In some cases, preventive measures such as avoiding triggers (such as bright lights or loud noises) or taking medications regularly can help to reduce the frequency of migraines.

The ketogenic diet is effective in reducing the frequency of migraines. In one study, people who followed a ketogenic diet for 3 months experienced significantly fewer migraines than those who did not follow the diet.

The ketogenic diet works by stabilizing blood sugar levels, which can help to prevent the changes in brain activity that are thought to trigger migraines. In addition, the diet helps to reduce inflammation, which is believed to play a role in the development of migraines.

In this beginner's guide, we'll discuss the following in detail:

- What are the types of migraines?
- What are the symptoms of migraine?
- What causes migraine?
- What are the risk factors for migraine?
- Migraine and women.
- How are migraines diagnosed?
- What are the medical treatments for migraine?
- What are the alternative treatments for migraine?
- How to prevent migraine?
- Managing migraine through natural methods and lifestyle changes.
- Managing migraine through a ketogenic diet.

If you want to learn more about how the ketogenic diet can help to manage migraines, read on.

Table of Contents

WHAT ARE THE TYPES OF MIGRAINES?

Migraines can be divided into two main types: migraine with aura and migraine without aura.

Migraine with aura: Migraine with aura, also known as classic migraine, is characterized by a warning sign or symptom (aura) that occurs before the headache. Auras typically last for less than 60 minutes and can include visual disturbances, such as flashing lights or blind spots. Other types of aura include tingling in the hands or feet, weakness, or difficulty speaking.

Migraine without aura: Migraine without aura, also known as common migraine, is the most common type of migraine. It is characterized by headache pain but does not include an aura.

Other types of migraine also include:

Basilar artery migraine: Basilar artery migraines are a rare form of migraine that affects the basilar artery, which runs from the base of the brain to the back of the head. Symptoms of a basilar artery migraine include dizziness, vertigo, and tinnitus, as well as sensitivity to light and sound.

Basilar artery migraines are often mistaken for other conditions, such as Meniere's disease or vestibular migraines. The exact cause of basilar artery migraines is unknown, but they are thought to be related to changes in blood flow to the brain. Treatment for basilar artery migraines typically includes medication and lifestyle changes. In some cases, surgery may be necessary to correct the underlying condition.

Hemiplegic migraine: Hemiplegic migraine is a neurological disorder characterized by temporary paralysis of one side of the body. The paralysis may affect the face, arm, and leg on one side or may be confined to the face. A hemiplegic migraine attack typically lasts for a few hours, although some people may experience paralysis for several days. During an attack, some people also experience visual disturbances, such as blindness or floaters. In addition, many people have headache pain during a hemiplegic migraine attack.

While the exact cause of hemiplegic migraine is unknown, it is thought to be due to abnormalities in the brain's blood vessels. Treatment for hemiplegic migraine typically involves pain relief medication and rest. In some cases, patients may also need physical therapy to regain movement in their affected limbs.

Ice cream headache: Most people agree that people who get migraines, especially those who have really bad ones, are more likely to also get ice cream headaches. In one study, 85% of people who had migraines also had this type of headache. People who get migraines may only feel it on one side, and it may even cause a full-blown migraine in these people, though this is rare.

Even though we don't fully understand how it works, it's thought that the cold makes the blood vessels in the head constrict, which causes pain when the vessels open up again. Some people may get ice cream headaches when they are about to get migraines. If you get ice cream headaches often or they are very bad, you should talk to your doctor about ways to prevent migraines.

Retinal migraine: Retinal migraine is a condition that causes temporary vision loss or changes in your field of vision. This can happen in one or both eyes. You may also have other symptoms, such as pain behind your eyes, dizziness, or headache.

Retinal migraine is often mistaken for other conditions, such as migraines with aura or optical migraines. It's important to see a doctor get a proper diagnosis. There is no specific treatment for retinal migraine, but you can manage your symptoms with medication and lifestyle changes.

Status migrainosus: Status migrainosus is a rare and potentially debilitating type of migraine headache that lasts for more than 72 hours. The exact cause is unknown, but it is believed to be triggered by a combination of factors, including hormonal changes, physical or emotional stress, or changes in sleep patterns. While the pain of status migrainosus can be severe, the condition itself is not life-threatening.

However, it can lead to other serious complications, such as dehydration and malnutrition. Treatment typically focuses on relieving the pain and preventing future episodes. In some cases, hospitalization may be required. With proper treatment, most people with status migrainosus can eventually return to their normal activities.

WHAT ARE THE SYMPTOMS OF MIGRAINE?

Migraine is a condition that causes severe head pain, often accompanied by other symptoms such as nausea, vomiting, and sensitivity to light and sound.

Headache: The pain of a migraine headache is usually throbbing or pulsing and is often on one side of the head. The pain may be moderate to severe.

Nausea: Many people with migraines also have nausea and vomiting.

Sensitivity to light and sound: Light and sound may aggravate or trigger migraine headaches in some people. This is why many people with migraines try to find a dark, quiet place to rest during an attack.

Aura: Some people with migraines also experience aura. Aura is a warning sign that a migraine is about to begin. It may include visual disturbances, such as flashes of light or blind spots, or tingling or numbness in the arm or leg.

What Causes Migraines?

Perhaps you've experienced it yourself: the intense headache that seems to come out of nowhere, accompanied by nausea, sensitivity to light and sound, and even dizziness. For many people, these symptoms are all too familiar, as they suffer from migraines regularly. While the exact cause of migraines is still unknown, there are several theories that scientists have come up with.

Change in brain activity: When a person has a migraine, the blood vessels in their brain constrict and then expand. This results in the release of chemicals that cause inflammation. The pain of a migraine is caused by the inflammation of the blood vessels and the pressure on the nerves.

Hormonal changes: It is well-known that women are more likely to experience migraines than men. Studies have shown that migraines are three times more common in women than in men. There are several theories about why this is the case, but one leading theory is that migraines are linked to hormonal changes. This theory is supported by the fact that women are more likely to experience migraines during times of hormonal changes, such as during puberty, pregnancy, and menopause.

While further research is needed to confirm this link, it is clear that hormones play a role in migraine development. As a result, women who suffer from migraines may need to take special precautions during times of hormonal changes.

Certain foods or drinks: In some cases, migraines may be caused by food sensitivities, so keeping a food journal can also help identify potential triggers. Some people find that certain foods or drinks trigger their migraines. Common triggers include aged cheeses, processed meats, chocolate, caffeine, and alcohol.

Sensory stimuli: Sensory stimuli are a common trigger for migraines. It is believed that certain sensory stimuli can cause changes in the brain, which in turn can trigger a migraine. Some of the most common triggers include bright lights, loud noises, and strong smells.

Changes in sleep: Migraine sufferers often report that their headaches start after a period of interrupted sleep or too little sleep. It's thought that these changes disrupt the body's natural rhythms, causing a cascade of events that leads to the formation of migraine headaches.

Stress: One of the most common triggers of migraines is stress. When a person experiences stress, their body goes into "fight or flight" mode, releasing hormones and chemicals that prepare them to deal with the perceived threat. While this response can be helpful in short-term situations, it can also lead to migraines when it is constantly activated.

People who experience chronic stress are more likely to suffer from migraines, and relaxation techniques can help to reduce the frequency and severity of migraine attacks. In addition, some research suggests that people who are prone to migraines may have a higher sensitivity to stress, making them more likely to experience headaches even under moderate amounts of stress.

Weather changes: Some people find that weather changes, such as barometric pressure changes, can trigger migraines.

Barometric pressure, humidity, and temperature can all affect the likelihood of a migraine. For example, barometric pressure drops before a storm, which can trigger headaches in susceptible people.

Similarly, high humidity levels can cause migraines by affecting the brain's electrical activity. While the exact mechanism is still not fully understood, it is clear that weather changes can be a migraine trigger for many people.

WHAT ARE THE RISK FACTORS FOR MIGRAINE?

Migraines are a common condition that can cause a variety of symptoms, including severe headaches, nausea, and sensitivity to light and sound. Although migraines can occur at any age, they are most common in adults. Several risk factors may increase your chances of developing migraines. These include family history, being female, certain lifestyle choices (such as smoking), and certain medical conditions (such as depression or anxiety).

Family history: One risk factor for migraine that is often overlooked is family history. If you have a family member who suffers from migraines, you are more likely to suffer from them as well. This is because migraines tend to run in families. Scientists believe that this may be due to genetics, although the exact mechanism is not yet understood. If you have a family history of migraines, it is important to be aware of the potential for developing them yourself.

Age: Age is a risk factor for migraine, with the risk increasing as you get older. The chance of having migraines starts to rise in childhood and adolescence, with the highest risk in adulthood. The risk then starts to decline after age 50.

There are several possible explanations for this increase in risk with age. One theory is that changes in hormone levels may play a role. Estrogen levels fluctuate during the menstrual cycle and decline after menopause, which may explain why migraines are more common in women than men.

Another possibility is that the aging process itself may lead to changes in the brain that make migraines more likely. Whatever the cause, age is an important risk factor for migraine that should be considered when evaluating your risk.

Gender: One risk factor for migraines is gender. Women are more likely than men to experience migraines. This may be due, in part, to hormonal changes. For example, migraine frequency has been found to increase during pregnancy and menstruation.

Additionally, women who take birth control pills or hormone replacement therapy may also be at increased risk for migraines. While the exact reasons for this link are not fully understood, it is clear that gender is a risk factor for migraine development. Therefore, women need to be aware of this and take steps to prevent migraines, such as identifying triggers and taking preventive medication.

Certain medical conditions: Migraines can be brought on by many different things. For some people, weather changes or certain foods can set off a migraine. Others have migraines that seem to appear out of nowhere. However, it is also common for migraines to be linked to underlying health conditions. Some of the most common medical conditions that are associated with migraines include:

- **Thyroid problems:** An overactive or underactive thyroid gland can cause a change in hormone levels, which can trigger migraines.
- **Sleep disorders:** Disruptions in sleep patterns can lead to migraines, especially if you are not getting enough restful sleep.
- **Depression:** It is thought that depression and migraines share a common neurological pathway, which is why migraines are often seen in people who suffer from depression.
- **Anxiety:** Like depression, anxiety is also linked to changes in brain chemistry that can trigger migraines.

If you suffer from frequent migraines, it is important to consult with a doctor to rule out any underlying health conditions. Treating the underlying condition can often help to reduce the frequency and intensity of migraines.

If you have any of these risk factors, it's important to talk to your doctor about your options for preventing or managing migraines. With the right treatment plan, you can minimize your symptoms and enjoy a more comfortable life.

MIGRAINES AND WOMEN

Migraine headaches are far more common in women than in males. In women of reproductive age across the world, migraine is the third most prevalent ailment that they suffer from. There are several potential migraine triggers, some of which include stress, hormonal changes, certain foods or chemicals, and others like these. The precise etiology of migraines is unclear. A significant number of women experience an increase in the frequency and severity of their migraines during menstruation and pregnancy.

Migraine headaches affect around 75 percent of all women and 25 percent of all males. Women between the ages of 20 and 45 are the demographic most likely to experience the debilitating effects of migraines. Women often have a higher amount of obligations in their careers, families, and communities as they reach this stage in their life.

Women are more likely to report headaches that are more intense and that continue for longer periods, in addition to experiencing other symptoms such as nausea and vomiting. When a woman suffers from a migraine, all of these factors combine to make it difficult for her to fulfill her obligations at both her place of employment and her home.

A migraine is a sickness that may be quite debilitating, but some therapies can help alleviate some of the symptoms. If you are a woman who suffers from migraines, you must discuss your treatment choices with your primary care physician. You should be able to lessen the severity of your symptoms and lead a life that is more pleasant if you choose the appropriate treatment strategy.

HOW MIGRAINES ARE DIAGNOSED?

If you suffer from migraines, it is important to consult your doctor. Be sure to write down the following information before your appointment:

- Your headache frequency.
- When headaches occur, such as during your period.
- Nausea or blind spots.
- A migraine-prone ancestor.
- All the prescription and over-the-counter drugs you take (better still, bring the medicines in their containers to the doctor).
- All the drugs you can remember taking, the dosages, and any negative effects.

At the appointment, your doctor will likely examine you and inquire about your health history. Past head injuries, and sinus or dental issues are examples. Your doctor may diagnose migraine from your symptoms. If your doctor suspects another cause, you may receive a blood test, CT scan, or MRI. Discuss the appropriate testing with your doctor.

WHAT ARE THE MEDICAL TREATMENTS FOR MIGRAINE?

There are two main types of medical treatment for migraines. These are the preventive medications and the acute medications.

Preventive medications: Preventive medications are a type of medical treatment for migraine that are taken regularly to try to reduce the number of migraine attacks a person experiences. These medications can be used alone or in combination with other treatments.

There are several types of preventive medications that are used to treat migraine, and they work in different ways. Preventives can be taken daily or just on days when a person is likely to have a migraine attack.

Some of the preventive medications include:

- **Calcium channel blockers:** Calcium channel blockers, such as verapamil, can help prevent migraines.
- **Beta-blockers:** Beta-blockers, such as propranolol, can help prevent migraines.

- **Botox:** Injections of botulinum toxin (Botox) can help prevent migraines.
- **Anticonvulsants:** Anticonvulsants, such as topiramate, can help prevent migraines.

They may need to be taken for several weeks or months before their full effects are seen. Side effects are different for each person, but they may include fatigue, dry mouth, weight gain, and low blood pressure. Preventive medications can sometimes help people with migraines who haven't been helped by other treatments. If you're considering taking preventive medication for your migraines, talk to your doctor about the risks and benefits to see if it's right for you.

Acute medications: Many different medications can be used to treat the symptoms of a migraine. Acute medications are those that are taken at the onset of a migraine to relieve the pain and other symptoms. Some of these acute medications are the following:

- **Over-the-counter pain relievers**: Over-the-counter (OTC) pain relievers, such as ibuprofen, can help relieve the pain of a migraine.
- **Ergotamines:** Ergotamines, such as Cafergot and Migergot, can help relieve the pain of migraine by narrowing the blood vessels around the brain, which helps to reduce the inflammation and pain associated with a migraine.
- **Triptans:** Triptans are a class of drugs that act on serotonin receptors in the brain. They are available in oral, nasal, and injectable forms.

- **Dopamine antagonists:** Dopamine antagonists, such as prochlorperazine, can help relieve nausea and vomiting associated with migraines.

If you are suffering from migraines, it is important to talk to your doctor about your treatment options.

WHAT ARE THE ALTERNATIVE TREATMENTS FOR MIGRAINE?

In addition to medical treatments, several alternative treatments may help relieve the symptoms of migraines.

Acupuncture: Since ancient times, people have turned to traditional Chinese medicine to treat a wide range of illnesses and conditions. One of the most well-known therapies is called acupuncture. It consists of putting very tiny needles into the skin of the patient at various places all over the body.

After receiving acupuncture therapy for their migraines, some patients report feeling alleviation from their symptoms. When carried out by a qualified professional, acupuncture is not only not thought to pose any health risks, but it also has the potential to be an efficient therapy choice for those who suffer from migraines.

Biofeedback: Biofeedback is a form of mind-body treatment that involves the use of sensors to monitor different processes of the body, such as the heart rate and the tension in the muscles. The purpose of biofeedback is to teach you how to exercise control over these activities of your body. Migraine sufferers may find relief from their symptoms with the use of biofeedback.

Biofeedback is a useful treatment for migraines, particularly when utilized in conjunction with other forms of treatment. Migraine patients could benefit from biofeedback since it teaches them how to exert control over their body's reaction to stress. There is some evidence that biofeedback can help reduce both the frequency and severity of migraines.

Massage: People who suffer from migraines may discover that getting massages help reduce their symptoms since it helps relax the muscles and releases tension. To do this, massage therapists employ several different methods, including kneading, tapping, and applying light, steady pressure on the client's head, neck, and shoulders. Even while further study is required to verify this claim, some people believe that getting frequent massages can help avoid migraines.

In addition to easing muscle tension and headaches, studies have shown that massage can also enhance circulation, promote immunity, and lower levels of stress. As a consequence of this, it should not come as a surprise that massage is increasingly being employed as an integral part of holistic medical practices.

Herbal remedies: Herbal treatments have been utilized for the treatment of a wide variety of disorders for many millennia. When it comes to finding treatment for migraines, ginger and feverfew are two of the most common herbs that are considered to be effective. However, there is little in the way of supporting evidence from the scientific community for their usage. Ginger has been the subject of several research studies, and those studies have shown conflicting results as to whether or not it might assist lessen the frequency and severity of migraines.

Regarding feverfew, a few more limited studies have revealed that it may help reduce the intensity of migraines; nevertheless, before any firm conclusions can be formed, bigger, more well-conducted trials are required. Therefore, herbal treatments may give some advantages to persons who suffer from migraines; nevertheless, further study is required to prove the usefulness of herbal remedies.

There is no treatment for migraines that is universally applicable to all patients. What works well for one individual might not be effective for another. It is essential to collaborate with your physician to develop the most effective treatment strategy for you.

MANAGING MIGRAINE THROUGH LIFESTYLE CHANGES

If you are one of the millions of individuals who suffer from migraines, then you are well aware of how incapacitating these headaches can be. It may be hard to work, interact with other people, or even take care of one's fundamental requirements if one is suffering from excruciating migraines, nausea, and sensitivity to light and sound.

Alterations to one's lifestyle, in addition to medical and alternative therapies, can be helpful in the management of migraines.

Getting enough sleep: The majority of people are aware that getting enough sleep each night is essential to maintaining general health; nevertheless, the significance of getting adequate sleep cannot be overstated for individuals who are afflicted by migraine headaches. Studies have shown that people with migraines tend to need 9-10 hours of sleep per night to feel fully rested and to reduce the frequency and severity of migraines. Even though getting this amount of sleep consistently might be challenging, migraine sufferers must make it one of their top priorities to do so.

Exercise: Exercising may be the last thing on the minds of many individuals who suffer from migraines since they associate it with painful symptoms. On the other hand, engaging in regular physical activity can help cut down on both the frequency and intensity of migraines. Exercise helps to enhance blood flow, which may help reduce pain, and it also helps to raise levels of endorphins, which can also help reduce pain.

In addition, physical activity can assist to lower levels of stress, which is a common factor in the development of migraines. Aim to complete at least 30 minutes of moderate exercise on most days of the week to achieve the best outcomes. Taking a stroll, riding a bike, or going for a swim are all excellent choices. And if you're worried that you won't be able to get in a whole 30 minutes at once, don't be; spreading it out over the day into three 10-minute sessions can also do the work.

Stress management: Migraines may be brought on by stress, which is common knowledge. However, many individuals are unaware that stress can also contribute to the severity and frequency of migraines. Mastering stress management techniques will help you cut down on the frequency of migraine attacks you suffer.

Yoga, meditation, and tai chi are just a few of the stress-relieving activities that are known to be particularly helpful. You might want to give some relaxation techniques like deep breathing or progressive muscle relaxation a go as well.

If you notice that you are constantly stressed, you should probably think about seeing a therapist or going to counseling. If you devote a portion of each day to activities that promote relaxation and stress management, you may be able to reduce the negative effects of stress on your life and migraines.

Avoiding triggers: Keeping a migraine diary can be a good approach to tracking your headaches and uncovering potential factors that may be causing them. The inability to get enough sleep, emotional stress, exposure to intense light, and consumption of particular foods are all common migraine triggers. You may be able to lessen the frequency of your migraines as well as their intensity if you steer clear of the causes listed above.

The ketogenic diet: There is some evidence that following a ketogenic diet can help reduce both the frequency and intensity of migraine headaches. A diet that is rich in fat and low in carbohydrates, known as the ketogenic diet, compels the body to use fat as its primary source of fuel.

If you're having trouble finding relief from your migraines, a conversation with your primary care physician is a good place to start. You might be able to decrease the influence that they have on your life with a little bit of work on your part.

MANAGING MIGRAINES THROUGH THE KETOGENIC DIET

A ketogenic diet is rich in fat, has a moderate amount of protein, and is low in carbs. This type of diet encourages the body to use fat for fuel rather than carbohydrates. The ketogenic diet was first designed as a method for treating epilepsy in children; however, recent research has revealed that it may also be beneficial in the treatment of diabetes, cancer, and weight reduction.

The ketogenic diet is effective because it weans the body off of glucose as a source of energy and teaches the metabolism to focus on the burning of fat rather than glucose. This metabolic state, known as ketosis, results in an accumulation of ketones in the blood, which, as previously mentioned, may provide several health advantages.

In addition to facilitating weight reduction and enhancing one's ability to maintain stable blood sugar levels, studies have shown that following a ketogenic diet can shield the brain against the onset of degenerative illnesses, lower levels of inflammation, and increase one's energy levels.

What to Eat on a Ketogenic Diet

The ketogenic diet is characterized by a high-fat content and a reduced emphasis on carbohydrates. On a ketogenic diet, you are permitted to consume items such as these:

Meat: Meat is an essential ingredient in the ketogenic diet and is considered one of its mainstays. Ketone bodies, which are utilized by the body as a source of energy, can be obtained through eating meat. Additionally, meat is an excellent source of protein as well as fat, all of which are necessary components of a healthy diet. On the ketogenic diet, acceptable cuts of meat include beef, hog, lamb, chicken, turkey, and others.

Fat: Increasing the amount of fat in one's diet by consuming foods like butter, ghee, lard, olive oil, and coconut oil is one way to facilitate the metabolic state of ketosis.

Fish: Fish like salmon, trout, tuna, and mackerel are all fantastic sources of healthy fats and protein, which makes them ideal for individuals who are following a ketogenic diet. In addition, fish is loaded with nutrients such as omega-3 fatty acids, which have been found to boost not just the health of the heart and brain but also a variety of other bodily functions.

Eggs: Consuming eggs in whole, including the yolk, is one of the fundamental tenets of the diet. The majority of an egg's nutrients, such as vitamins A, D, and E, as well as choline and lutein, are contained in the yolk of the egg. Other nutrients found in yolk include: The egg yolk also has a higher concentration of fat than the egg white, which is essential for individuals following the ketogenic diet because fat is one of the primary dietary sources of energy.

Vegetables: The ketogenic diet places a strong emphasis on the consumption of vegetables. They have low carbohydrate and calorie content, but a high concentration of beneficial elements such as vitamins, minerals, and antioxidants. Vegetables provide fiber, which is an essential component for maintaining digestive health and warding against constipation. Because of these factors, increasing the number of veggies in your diet is one of the best things you can do for your health.

Fruits: Studies conducted on animals have indicated that following a ketogenic diet can both improve cognitive performance and extend lifespan. The consumption of fruits that contain healthy fats, such as avocados, coconuts, and berries, can assist in the promotion of the aforementioned advantages. Additionally, these fruits are an excellent source of the vitamins, minerals, and fiber that are necessary for maintaining a healthy body. You can increase the likelihood of the ketogenic diet's positive effects on your health by eating a diet that contains the fruits listed here.

Nuts and seeds: Incorporating nuts and seeds into your diets, such as almonds, walnuts, and pumpkin seeds, amongst other options, is an excellent way to obtain a source of healthy fats that may assist you in meeting your daily fat consumption objectives. Incorporating these items into your diet not only contributes to the maintenance of excellent health but also helps to boost the diversity of nutrients that you take in via your eating habits. In addition, nuts and seeds are an excellent source of fiber, which is useful for digestion and assists in maintaining a sense of fullness for a longer period.

Dairy: However, dairy products have a very high carbohydrate content despite being an important source of calcium. As a direct consequence of this, the keto diet encourages its followers to completely abstain from consuming any dairy products. On the other hand, some dairy products are OK to consume when following a ketogenic diet.

People who are attempting to adhere completely to the diet might benefit by consuming full-fat milk, yogurt, and cheese because all three of these dairy products have relatively low carb counts. In addition, these meals include a high quantity of other nutrients that are necessary for maintaining a healthy body, such as vitamin D and protein. On the ketogenic diet, dairy products can be beneficial so long as the consumption of these items is kept within reasonable limits.

What to Avoid on a Ketogenic Diet

A ketogenic diet is high in fat, moderate in protein, and low in carbohydrates. When adhering to this diet, it is essential to stay away from meals that contain a high concentration of carbs.

Grains: The body converts the starch found in grains into glucose, which is then utilized for energy. Grains contain a significant quantity of starch. However, if the intake of carbs is limited, the body will be forced to seek alternative sources of energy. This can be accomplished by converting the body's stored fat into ketones, which are then utilized as a source of fuel by the brain as well as other tissues. Therefore, if you are following a ketogenic diet, limiting grains is one of the most effective ways to enhance ketosis and weight reduction.

Starchy vegetables: It is essential to stay away from starchy foods like potatoes, sweet potatoes, carrots, and other root vegetables when adhering to a ketogenic diet. Because of the high carbohydrate content of certain veggies, eating them may cause you to get kicked out of ketosis and hinder you from attaining the outcomes you want from the diet.

Fruit: If you are following a ketogenic diet, you should stay away from specific fruits including apples, oranges, bananas, and any other fruits that are rich in sugar content. Even though these fruits may be beneficial for certain people's health, eating them might cause your blood sugar levels to spike fast and take you out of ketosis.

Stick to low-sugar fruits such as berries, which are also strong in antioxidants and other healthy elements. Berries are a good example of this. You will be able to stay on track with your ketogenic diet and enjoy all of the health benefits that come along with it if you steer clear of these high-sugar fruits.

Sugar: Avoid consuming meals that may cause an increase in your insulin levels and prevent you from entering ketosis if you are following a ketogenic diet. This will help you stay in ketosis longer. Because of this, it is essential to steer clear of consuming sweet foods such as honey, agave syrup, or maple syrup in any form. These meals not only include sugar, which can drive you out of ketosis, but they also contain empty calories, which can lead to weight gain. This means that eating these foods can cause you to gain weight.

Processed foods: Following a ketogenic diet is associated with several health advantages, some of which include weight loss, enhanced mental clarity, and reduced inflammation. On the other hand, if you want to get these benefits, you need to stay away from processed meals. This is because processed foods include a large number of carbs, which, if consumed, might force your body out of ketosis and prevent you from experiencing the full therapeutic effects of the diet.

It has been demonstrated that following a ketogenic diet, which is high in fat and low in carbohydrates, can help lessen the frequency and intensity of migraine headaches. The ketogenic diet is effective because it tricks the body into using fat as fuel rather than carbs. This brings to a metabolic condition known as ketosis, which has a role in reducing inflammation and discomfort.

If you are considering giving the ketogenic diet a shot, you must see a medical professional or a qualified dietitian to devise a meal strategy that is tailored to your specific needs.

SAMPLE RECIPES

Baked Flounder

Ingredients:

- 1 lb. flounder, fileted
- 1/4 tsp. salt
- 1 tbsp. extra-virgin olive oil
- 2 tbsp. parsley, chopped finely
- 1 cup almonds, chopped and toasted
- freshly ground black pepper, to taste

Instructions:

1. Preheat the oven to 375°F.
2. Place fish on a sheet tray. Season with olive oil, salt, and pepper.
3. Combine the almonds, grapes, parsley, 1-1/2 tsp. of olive oil, 1/8 tsp of salt, and black pepper in a bowl.
4. Bake the fish for about 3 minutes.
5. Flip the fish and return it to the oven.
6. Bake for another 3 minutes, or until the fish is starting to flake, while the center is still translucent. Don't overcook.

7. Serve immediately.

Chicken Salad

Ingredients:

- 1 small can of premium chunk chicken breast packed in water
- 1 stalk celery, large, finely chopped
- 1/4 cup reduced-fat mayonnaise
- 4 romaine leaves or red leaf lettuce, washed and trimmed
- 1 cucumber, small and sliced thinly

Instructions:

1. Drain canned chicken and transfer to a bowl.
2. Put in celery and mayonnaise.
3. Mix lightly. Don't crush the chicken.
4. In a separate shallow bowl, place the lettuce neatly.
5. Add the chicken salad in the middle
6. Add cucumber slices to the plate.
7. Refrigerate before serving, cover with plastic wrap.

Baked Salmon

Ingredients:

- 2 salmon filets
- 6 cups of fresh spinach
- 2 tsp. coconut oil
- 1/4 tsp. turmeric

- salt
- pepper

Instructions:

1. Preheat the oven to 400°F.
2. Line a baking dish with parchment paper.
3. Marinate salmon filets coconut oil, turmeric, salt, and pepper.
4. Let it sit for a few minutes. This may also be done the night before to help the juices and flavor get into the salmon.
5. Once the oven is ready, bake salmon for 15 minutes.
6. Add spinach and cook until ready. Season with salt and pepper to taste.
7. Take salmon out of the oven and put spinach beside it.
8. Serve and enjoy.

Asparagus and Greens Salad with Tahini and Poppy Seed Dressing

Ingredients:

- 10 to 12 asparagus stalks, washed well and sliced into ribbons
- 5 radishes, washed well, and sliced thinly
- 2 to 3 rainbow carrots, peeled and sliced thinly
- 1 handful of wild spinach
- 1 small handful of microgreens, washed well
- 1 small handful of sunflower greens, washed well
- optional: a few pieces of chive blossoms

For the dressing:

- 2 tbsp. tahini
- 1 tbsp. poppy seeds
- 1 tbsp. extra-virgin olive oil
- salt
- pepper

Instructions:

1. For the dressing, whisk ingredients together in a small bowl.
2. In a separate bowl, toss salad ingredients in the mixture.
3. Drizzle dressing on salad upon serving.

Roasted Chicken Thighs

Ingredients:

- 1 tbsp. avocado oil
- 1 pinch Himalayan pink salt
- 4 chicken thighs with skin
- 1 tsp. Primal Palate super gyro seasoning

Instructions:

1. Pour avocado oil over a medium-sized oven-safe pot.
2. Sauté over medium heat for 2 to 3 minutes or until the skins begin to brown.
3. Place the chicken in a large skillet over medium-high heat. Sear for about 2 to 3 minutes for each side, starting with the skin side.

4. Season generously with salt and Primal Palate Super Gyro seasoning.
5. Place the chicken in an oven preheated to 350°F.
6. Bake for one hour while covered.
7. Serve and enjoy.

Arugula and Mushroom Salad

Ingredients:

- 5 oz. arugula washed
- 1 lb. fresh mushrooms
- 1/4 tsp. shoyu
- 1 tbsp. olive oil
- 1 tbsp. mirin

For tofu cheese:

- 1/8 cup umeboshi vinegar
- 1/2 firm tofu

Instructions:

1. In a bowl, add the rinsed tofu. Crumble and pour in vinegar.
2. In a separate bowl add shoyu, salt, olive oil, and mirin. 3. Mix to combine.
3. Add in the arugula and toss to combine with the dressing.
4. Serve and enjoy.

Fresh Asparagus Salad

Ingredients:

- 1/3 cup of hazelnuts
- 4 cups arugula
- 1 tsp. ground pepper
- 2 tbsp. sea salt
- virgin olive oil
- 2 lbs. asparagus

Instructions:

1. Preheat the oven to 400°F.
2. Place hazelnuts on a baking tray with parchment paper. Place in the oven for 7 minutes.
3. Transfer hazelnuts to a plate. Optionally, to remove the skins, wrap the nuts in a towel and rub them vigorously.
4. Chop hazelnuts coarsely.
5. Remove the hard ends of the asparagus.
6. Place the stalks on the baking sheet you've used for the hazelnuts. Sprinkle 1 tbsp. olive oil and 1/2 tsp. of salt.
7. Bake for 8 minutes.
8. In a mixing bowl, combine pepper, salt, and olive oil. Mix well.
9. Place the arugula in a medium bowl. Drizzle half of the dressing over the veggies. Toss until everything is well coated.
10. Place arugula onto a platter.
11. Arrange asparagus on top. Sprinkle peeled hazelnuts on top.

Tuna Salad

Ingredients:

- 1/2 cup pecans
- 1 cup chicken breast, steamed and cubed
- 1 cup tuna in oil
- salt, to taste
- pepper, to taste

Instructions:

1. Mix all ingredients in a large bowl.
2. Add a dash of salt and pepper to taste.
3. Chill for at least an hour before serving.

Baked Chicken Breasts

Ingredients:

For the chicken breast:

- 4 chicken breasts, boneless and skinless
- 1 tbsp. olive oil
- 4 cups lukewarm water

For the chicken seasoning blend:

- 1/2 tsp. paprika, sweet or smoked
- 1/4 tsp. salt
- 1/4 tsp. fresh ground pepper

- 1/2 tsp. garlic powder
- 1/8 tsp. pepper
- 1/2 tsp. onion powder
- 1/2 tsp. dried thyme
- 1/2 tsp. dried rosemary
- 1/4 tsp. parsley, dried or fresh, chopped, for garnish

Instructions:

1. Preheat the oven to 425°F.
2. Combine lukewarm water and salt in a large bowl.
3. Add the chicken breasts. Leave for 20 to 30 minutes.
4. In a separate container, combine the dry ingredients of the seasoning blend with a fork.
5. Pour out the salt water. Rinse each chicken breast under cold water. Dry.
6. Place the chicken in a baking dish and rub olive oil all over.
7. Evenly apply seasoning blend over the chicken on all sides.
8. Place in the oven to cook for 22 to 25 minutes. Check if the internal temperature reaches 165°F.
9. Make sure to keep an eye on the breasts, as each piece may cook faster than the rest.
10. Broil the chicken until the top parts are golden.
11. If you want a browned and crispier top, set the oven to broil on high for the final 4 minutes.
12. Transfer to a serving plate to rest for 10 minutes before cutting.
13. Garnish with parsley upon serving.

Steak with Olive Oil

Ingredients:

- 2 8-oz. grass-fed New York strip steaks, about 1-1/2-inch-thick, trimmed
- 3 tbsp. olive oil, divided
- 1 tsp. freshly ground black pepper, divided
- 1 tsp. kosher salt, divided
- 1 garlic clove, crushed
- 1 rosemary sprig
- optional: rosemary leaves

Instructions:

1. Place the grill pan over medium-high heat.
2. Brush a tablespoon of oil on the steak, then sprinkle with half a teaspoon of salt and another half teaspoon of pepper.
3. Put a tablespoon of oil into the pan, followed by a rosemary sprig and garlic.
4. Cook steak for about 9 minutes, or until preferred doneness is achieved. For every minute, turn the steak and baste it with oil.
5. Transfer the steak to a cutting board, letting it rest for 5 minutes.
6. Slice steak across the grain and place it on a platter. Drizzle with the juice from the cutting board and the leftover oil.
7. Sprinkle it with the remaining salt and pepper.
8. Upon serving, garnish with rosemary leaves if desired.

Beef Heart

Ingredients:

- 1 tbsp. ghee
- 4 slices beef heart, about an inch thick
- 2 tbsp. olive oil, rosemary-infused or plain
- salt
- pepper*

Instructions:

1. Take heart slices from the marinade and pat dry.
2. Heat a cast-iron skillet with the ghee on a high flame for 2-3 minutes.
3. Lay the meat in the skillet. The temperature should be high enough to sizzle.
4. Cook for 5 minutes on each side until nicely browned on the outside but still pink in the middle.
5. Drizzle with rosemary-infused olive oil.
6. Serve with a salad of choice.

*black pepper may be substituted with white pepper

Grilled Lamb

Ingredients:

- 1-1/2 lb. baby spinach leaves
- 3 tbsp. dried oregano, chopped
- 1/4 cup lemon juice
- 1/4 cup olive oil

- 2 tbsp. ground cumin
- 1 tsp. crushed red pepper
- 1 tbsp. coarse sea salt
- 1 tbsp. squeezed juice from an orange
- 3 cloves of garlic
- 2 yellow onions, chopped
- cooking spray

Instructions:

1. In a 2-gallon zip bag, put the lamb together with the lemon juice, oregano, cumin, and salt.
2. Close the bag and refrigerate overnight
3. Puree onions, garlic, some orange juice, and olive oil in a blender.
4. Transfer to a small bowl with a cover.
5. Chill overnight.
6. Mix sea salt, red pepper, and cumin in a small bowl
7. Remove refrigerated lamb and let it sit for 30 minutes.
8. Preheat the grill to medium.
9. Place lamb on the grill and coat with some cooking spray or oil.
10. Grill lamb for one and a half hours over medium heat.
11. Remove the lamb from the grill.
12. Serve hot.

Conclusion

Migraines are a specific kind of headache that frequently manifest themselves alongside additional symptoms, such as sensitivity to light and sound as well as nausea and vomiting. A migraine headache can be quite painful and make it difficult to go about your everyday activities.

There are many different kinds of migraines, and each one has its unique collection of symptoms. The classical migraine, which is the most frequent kind of migraine and is preceded by an aura, is also the most severe type of migraine. Other kinds of migraines include the following:

- basilar artery migraine
- hemiplegic migraine
- ice cream headache
- retinal migraine
- status migrainosus

Migraines may strike anybody, although women are more likely than males to suffer from them. It is not completely understood what causes migraines, although it is believed that several variables, including genetics, environment, and lifestyle choices, are involved in their development.

Stress, smoking, drinking alcohol, not getting enough sleep, and hormonal shifts are some of the things that might put you at risk for suffering migraines. Because migraine symptoms can differ from person to person, diagnosing migraines can be challenging. Taking a comprehensive medical history and doing a thorough physical exam are the two most typical steps in diagnosing migraines.

There are several medical therapies available for migraines, such as prescription drugs and injections. Additionally, there are several natural remedies, such as making adjustments to one's lifestyle and utilizing a ketogenic diet.

Migraines may be managed most effectively by preventative measures, and several things can be done to lower the likelihood of acquiring migraines. These include lowering stress levels, getting adequate sleep, avoiding triggers, and utilizing a ketogenic diet. One such diet is known as the ketogenic diet, and it consists of eating a lot of fat and very few carbs. For some people, this is a useful method for preventing and treating migraines.

References

Ball, D. J., M.S., & RD. (n.d.). Complete Keto Diet Food List: What You Can and Cannot Eat If You're on a Ketogenic Diet. EatingWell. Retrieved September 22, 2022, from https://www.eatingwell.com/article/291245/complete-keto-diet-food-list-what-you-can-and-cannot-eat-if-youre-on-a-ketogenic-diet/.

Foods to Avoid on a Ketogenic Diet [Complete List]. (2018, October 14). Ruled Me. https://www.ruled.me/foods-to-avoid-on-a-ketogenic-diet-what-is-keto-friendly/.

How to Add More Fiber to Your Diet. (n.d.). Mayo Clinic. Retrieved September 22, 2022, from https://www.mayoclinic.org/healthy-lifestyle/nutrition-and-healthy-eating/in-depth/fiber/art-20043983.

Is a Keto Diet Helpful for Migraines and Cluster Headaches? (n.d.). Diet Doctor. Retrieved September 22, 2022, from https://www.dietdoctor.com/low-carb/migraines-cluster-headaches.

Masood, W., Annamaraju, P., & Uppaluri, K. R. (2022). Ketogenic Diet. In StatPearls. StatPearls Publishing. http://www.ncbi.nlm.nih.gov/books/NBK499830/.

Migraine | Office on Women's Health. (n.d.). Retrieved September 22, 2022, from https://www.womenshealth.gov/a-z-topics/migraine.

Migraine. (2017, October 23). NHS.uk. https://www.nhs.uk/conditions/migraine/.

What Causes Ice Cream Headaches? (n.d.). Scientific American. Retrieved September 22, 2022, from https://www.scientificamerican.com/article/what-causes-ice-cream-hea/.

9 798868 915666